The Blood Type Diet

Revealed: A Healthy Way To Eat Right And Lose Weight Based On Your Blood Type

Copyright 2015 by Better Life Solutions- All rights reserved.

This document is geared towards providing exact and reliable information in regards to the topic and issue covered. The publication is sold with the idea that the publisher is not required to render accounting, officially permitted, or otherwise, qualified services. If advice is necessary, legal or professional, a practiced individual in the profession should be ordered.

- From a Declaration of Principles which was accepted and approved equally by a Committee of the American Bar Association and a Committee of Publishers and Associations.

In no way is it legal to reproduce, duplicate, or transmit any part of this document in either electronic means or in printed format. Recording of this publication is strictly prohibited and any storage of this document is not allowed unless with written permission from the publisher. All rights reserved.

The information provided herein is stated to be truthful and consistent, in that any liability, in terms of inattention or otherwise, by any usage or abuse of any policies, processes, or directions contained within is the solitary and utter responsibility of the recipient reader. Under no circumstances will any legal responsibility or blame be held against the publisher for any reparation, damages, or monetary loss due to the information herein, either directly or indirectly.

Respective authors own all copyrights not held by the publisher.

The information herein is offered for informational purposes solely, and is universal as so. The presentation of the information is without contract or any type of guarantee assurance.

The trademarks that are used are without any consent, and the publication of the trademark is without permission or backing by the trademark owner. All trademarks and brands within this book are for clarifying purposes only and are the owned by the owners themselves, not affiliated with this document.

Table of Contents

Introduction 4

Chapter 1 – The importance of the blood type 5

Chapter 2 – What is the blood type diet? 10

Chapter 3 – The blood type A diet 15

Chapter 4 – The blood type B diet 22

Chapter 5 – The blood type O diet... 28

Chapter 6 – The blood type AB diet 34

Conclusion..41

Introduction

This book contains proven steps and strategies on how to eat healthy and lose weight based on your blood type.

If you are interested in discovering everything there is to know about the blood type diet, this guide is the essential resource for you to read. It will teach you the healthy eating choices for losing weight, based on your blood type.

Here Is A Preview Of What You'll Learn...

- The importance of the blood type for your health
- What is the blood type diet
- The blood type A diet foods
- The blood type B diet foods
- The blood type O diet foods
- The blood type AB diet foods
- How to take advantage of your genetic inheritance and lose weight
- Foods you should avoid according to your blood type

Much, much more!

Chapter 1 – The importance of the blood type

The blood type is an essential element for the health of the human body, transmitting the genetic inheritance from our ancestors and influencing our overall well-being. Today, due to the extensive research in the field, it is known that the blood type has a definite influence on the health of different organs and systems in the body. For example, the blood type can determine if a person will be successful or not in losing weight. This is the reason why knowing your blood type can actually help you better understand your body, including when it comes to the following aspects: reaction to different types of food, susceptibility to certain illnesses and the stress response.

Scientists have managed to demonstrate that each blood type comes with a higher risk for developing certain conditions, the same blood type having a low risk for other afflictions. For example, the people who have the O blood type are known to present a low susceptibility to cardiovascular problems, while the risk for developing stomach ulcers is high. Those who have the A blood type may develop microbial infections in a higher percentage than other people but it is the blood type that guarantees their high rate of fertility (valid for women who have this blood type). On the other hand, those who have the B and AB blood types are more prone to developing certain types of cancer, including pancreatic cancer.

As it was already mentioned, the blood type also determines the stress response, which, in its turn, can influence the overall health and also the capacity of losing weight. In people who have the A blood type, the levels of cortisol hormones are higher than in people who have other blood types, these levels increasing even further in case of a stressful situation. On the other hand, those who have the O blood type are known to have the 'fight or flight' response to stress. Basically, their body reacts to a stressful situation by producing higher quantities of adrenaline. While this might help them out of a stressful situation, it also means that they need a longer period of time to recover from the respective situation.

The antigens that are specific for each blood type are not found just in the blood but also in other parts of the body, including at the level of the digestive tract. This means that the blood type antigens have a definite influence on the way the body interacts with the food that you are eating. For example, the lectins that are contained in certain foods can easily bind to the blood type antigens and lead to the agglutination of the blood. When such a thing happens, the physical symptoms you might experience include a state of general weakness, accompanied by headaches and digestive complaints. Your skin can also be affected by eating foods that are incompatible with your blood type (reading that, you can certainly understand that, by choosing the right foods, you can also have a beautiful skin).

Keep in mind that the blood type also has an influence over the intestinal bacteria and the way it decomposes food. The type-A blood type is known to break down carbohydrates efficiently, using it for energy. On the other hand, the type-O blood type transforms the carbs into fat deposits, as opposed to breaking them down. This might suggest that each person, according to his/her blood type, has nutritional needs that are different. Using the blood type to determine these nutritional needs is the basis of the blood type diet, allowing you to lose weight, reduce the inflammation in different parts of the body and feel more energetic.

As you will see in the next chapter, the blood type diet will teach you to choose foods that are compatible with your blood type, being low in lection and reducing the risk for different diseases you might be susceptible to. It will teach you what foods to eat and what foods you should avoid, providing useful information on the most important types of physical exercises that can be made (once more, according to your blood type).

The human body is a perfect machine and it functions alright, as long as it is properly maintained. Just like a machine, you need to learn to use the right fuel, in order for your body to function at an optimal level. If you want to be healthy and lose the extra weight, you should consider the foods that you eat and the chemical reactions that occur inside your body when you eat certain foods. You should always remember that your blood type makes you predisposed to certain dietary intolerances, such as the one to dairy products or the one to gluten.

There are many foods that are incompatible with your blood type, as you will have the opportunity to discover in the following chapters. In the majority of these cases, the foods contain lectins that come from different protein sources. These, as it was already explained, bind to the blood antigen and lead to all sort of health problems, affecting the liver, stomach or other parts of the intestinal tract.

While it is true that you cannot do anything to change your blood type, this does not mean that you are doomed forever.

On the contrary, you can put all this information about your blood type to good use and change your diet today. As you will read below, the blood type diet has been designed so as to protect your genetic inheritance and teach you to choose only the foods that are compatible with your blood type antigens. If you decide to take your blood type into consideration, you will have a healthy intestinal flora and also reduce the risk of developing certain medical problems in the future. You will definitely enjoy the renewed levels of energy, losing all that extra weight and eliminating the abdominal discomfort you have experienced in the past.

Let's find out more information on the blood type diet and

how it can help you improve your overall health, promoting a state of well-being!

Chapter 2 – What is the blood type diet?

The blood type diet is based on the idea that the blood type can be used in order to determine the diet choices that are healthy. Proposed by Peter J. D'Adamo, this diet includes different food choices for each blood type. As it was mentioned in the above chapter, this diet stems from the idea that people digest the lectins in various types of foods differently. According to this proposer of this theory, each blood type has an antigen marker that is unique. In eating foods that are not compatible with the blood type, the antigen binds to the food and leads to a wide range of health problems. On the other hand, by eating the foods that are compatible with the blood type, one can stay healthy and lose weight in a manner that is 100% efficient.

It is said that our evolutionary heritage is hidden in our blood types. This means that each blood type should consume the foods our ancestors used to eat. For example, those who have the O-blood type are considered to be part of the ancestral blood group, which means that their diet should primarily include animal proteins. These are the kind of people who also benefit from intense physical exercise – in order to lose weight, they should consider aerobics, jogging, running, contact sports and even martial arts. In terms of diet, they should avoid dairy products and the sources of gluten (such as wheat), as these contribute to their weight gain.

Those who have the A-blood type are considered to stem from the humans that formed settled communities, living on the food they used to cultivate. Their diet should be primarily vegetarian, with food choices that are fresh, pure and organic. As for the physical exercise, this should not be intense but rather calming, such as yoga or Tai Chi. The vegetarian diet can also help those in this blood group to reduce the risk for chronic conditions, including cardiovascular disease, diabetes or cancer.

The B-blood type group is considered to have descended from nomadic tribes, having most powerful immune system and a digestive system that is highly tolerant to varied types of foods. The people who have belong to this blood type should consume dairy products, as these can protect them against chronic and degenerative medical problems. In terms of physical exercise, this should be moderate, with hiking, swimming, tennis and cycling among the most suitable choices.

The AB-blood type is considered the most recent group and the most complex from a biological point of view. Those who have this blood type should consume foods recommended to those in the A and B blood groups, as they can benefit from this combo diet.

It is considered that the blood type diet can not only help you lose weight but also to reduce the risk of developing certain types of medical conditions. According to the developers of this diet, each blood group has a susceptibility to a wide range of medical problems. The O-type group is prone to respiratory problems and allergies, such as asthma and hay fever. It is also believed that this group presents an increased risk of developing arthritis, especially with the increased consumption of carbs (inflammatory process at the level of the joints).

The B-type group presents a high resistance to developing allergies but it can develop such problems by choosing the wrong types of food. Apart from that, they present an increased susceptibility to autoimmune disorders, including multiple sclerosis, systemic lupus erythematosus and chronic fatigue. Those who belong to the A-type group are known to develop cardiac problems, cancer or anemia. In the situation of the AB-type group, the susceptibility is increased to diabetes and cancer (negative prognosis when it comes to survival).

The blood type diet can be efficiently used for losing weight; as the proposers of this diet have shown, there seems to be a direct link between the blood type and the functioning of the digestive tract (especially when it comes to the stomach acidity and the enzymes involved in the digestion process). By following a diet that is suitable to your blood type, your body will digest food in a more efficient manner. This also means that the food is going to be absorbed and not deposited as fat. You will be able to lose weight and stay healthy for the rest of your life. Plus, you will certainly enjoy the fresh and natural foods that are recommended for your specific blood type. There is no junk food allowed in this diet, so you should prepare yourself for a lifestyle change as well.

In conclusion, this is not a diet per say but rather a way of living. You get to make healthy food choices, based on your blood type and enjoy the benefits offered, the weight loss being one of the most important. If you have always wanted to lose weight and none of the diets you have tried worked out, it is time to consider the diet choices recommended for your blood type.

Chapter 3 – The blood type A diet

Each of the four blood types has gone through a series of biological adaptations throughout time, one of the most important ones being related to the digestive structure. Those who are in the blood type A group are known to possess lower levels of hydrochloric acid in the stomach. Apart from that, it seems that the intestinal enzymes responsible for digestion are present in higher levels. Both these two adaptations contribute to the efficient breaking down of the carbs, these being used for energy. However, the levels of alkaline phosphatase in the intestine are low as well, which means that the persons in this blood group have trouble digesting proteins that come from animal sources.

Being part of a certain blood groups also means that you have a genetic predisposition to certain medical problems. The blood type A group is susceptible to developing different types of cancer, diabetes and cardiovascular disease. With the blood type diet, you can change your lifestyle, discovering foods that are beneficial for your health and exercises that are going to help you keep in shape as well. The choices made thanks to the blood type are going to change your way of living, improving your overall performance. You can say goodbye to the mental fog, experiencing a renewed clarity and vitality. All of these things are going to guarantee a long and healthy life.

The blood type A group benefits from a vegetarian diet and, as you will have the opportunity to see on your own, by eliminating meat and other toxic foods from your diet, you will finally be able to lose weight. At first, you may have a hard time switching from meals that are based on meat to other sources of proteins (such as soy), grains or vegetables. However, you should remember that the persons who have this type of blood are extremely sensitive and they benefit the most from food that is fresh and organic. By changing your diet and including more natural foods, you can improve the strength of your immune system and reduce the risk of chronic diseases.

No matter your blood type, you can acknowledge that we live in a word that is defined by stress. In regard to your specific blood type, those who are in the blood type A group are known to present high levels of cortisol, which is known as the stress hormone. When they are face to face with a stressful situation, the body responds by producing even more cortisol. The problem is that these elevated levels of cortisol can wreak havoc on the health of your body, disrupting your sleeping pattern and influencing your cognitive performance during the day (brain fog). The blood can become thicker (hence the risk for cardiovascular disease), not to mention the body consumes the muscular tissue and not the adipose one. In people who have abnormal levels of cortisol, more severe health problems can appear, including: diabetes due to insulin resistance, hypothyroidism due to the hormonal imbalances and different disorders, including obsessive-compulsive disorder.

You need to remember that the blood type diet requires a lot of changes to be made in regard to your lifestyle. If you want to keep the cortisol levels within the normal levels, you will have to limit your sugar intake, as well as give up caffeine and alcohol. You need to respect a strict meal schedule and never skip meals, especially breakfast. In order to keep the blood sugar at stable levels, you will have to get accustomed to eating meals that are smaller in size but more frequent throughout the day. It is also recommended that you avoid the situations in which the cortisol levels might increase, leading to mental exhaustion among other problems: extreme noises, violent movies, excessive emotions, smoking, not getting enough sleep, extreme temperatures, strong smells and working incessantly. Consuming high quantities of starch or sugar is also forbidden, as it can lead to a high increase in blood sugar levels, followed by a sudden crash.

The diet for the blood type A also includes a regular program of exercise – it is recommended that you try out the exercises that have a calming effect, avoiding those that are too intense. Among the recommended choices for physical activity, there are: Tai Chi, yoga, meditation and deep breathing.

Before we move on to the food list recommended for this blood type, there are a few things that you should remember about this lifestyle change. First of all, you will need to organize your daily schedule, so that you balance the work and relaxation time. It is recommended that you go to bed early and try to get at least eight hours of sleep. Apart from that, if you have a sedentary job, try to take frequent breaks. During these breaks, make sure that you get physically active – you can do a few stretching exercises, take a short walk or even do some deep breathing exercises. As it was already mentioned, do not skip meals, no matter how much work you might have to do. Also, it is recommended that the highest intake of protein is during the day, the quantity being reduced throughout the rest of the meals. During each meal, make sure that the food is thoroughly chewed, as this also promotes a better digestion and absorption process (blood type A group has reduced levels of hydrochloric acid in the stomach, which means that the digestion is slower).

As there is a very strong connection between anxiety and stress, avoid eating when you feel anxious (you might increase your cortisol levels even further). Accustom yourself to eating when you are relaxed, choosing meals that are smaller and increasing their frequency throughout the day. Never forget your calming exercises and try to perform them at least several times per week. In order to reduce the risk of chronic health problems, visit the doctor on a regular basis. Remember, it is always for the best to prevent rather than treat.

In regard to the actual foods to be included in the blood type A diet, you are allowed to eat plenty of fish, including salmon, trout, cod and mackerel. On the other hand, you should reduce your intake of chicken and poultry to maximum two times per week. It is recommended that you eliminate other types of meat from your diet, including shellfish, any type of game, pork and beef. Dairy products, including eggs, should be excluded as well but the good news is that you can use substitutes, such as rice or soy milk. Depending on your tolerance to lactose, there may some dairy products that you can consume, such as yogurt, kefir or different types of cheeses (most commonly, goat cheese).

The main types of foods that should be included in the blood type diet are fresh vegetables and fruits. In regard to the vegetables that you should consider consuming, these are the recommended choices: dark leafy greens (spinach, kale), collard greens, turnips, broccoli, onions and artichokes. As for the fruits, you are allowed to eat blueberries, grapefruits, pineapples, figs, cherries and plums. There are certain fruits and vegetables that are allowed to consume only occasionally, such as: apples, strawberries, beets, cucumbers, avocado and asparagus. The fruits and vegetables that you should take off from the list include: oranges, bananas, potatoes, tomatoes, eggplants and cabbages.

In terms of grains, you are allowed to consume sprouted wheat and cereals, such as buckwheat and kasha. You can also add different types of flour to your diet, including rice, rye and oat flour. White flour, made from wheat and semolina should be avoided. For one or two times a week, you can consume the following products: quinoa, couscous, corn, barley and rice. Pumpkin seeds and peanuts are accepted and so are peas and different types of beans (however, you should avoid navy and kidney types).

Pistachios and cashews are not accepted, so these should be excluded as well.

For eating and cooking, you are allowed to use both olive and flaxseed oil. The moderate consumption of other types of oil is accepted, including cod liver and canola oil. The oils that you should avoid include: corn, sesame, safflower and peanut. In regard to spices and condiments, you can use the following: mustard, garlic, ginger, miso, tamari and soy sauce. Pickles, different salad dressings and jam (made from recommended fruits) should be consumed in moderation. Among the things that you should exclude from your diet, there are: ketchup, mayo, pepper and vinegar.

As you can see, there are certain foods that you are allowed to eat and others that have to be excluded from the diet. If you follow these recommendations, you will definitely lose all that extra weight in a short amount of time.

Chapter 4 – The blood type B diet

Those who have the blood type B are known to come from nomad ancestors, whose diet consisted primarily of meat and dairy. They are known to respond to stress by producing increased quantities of cortisol and they also present a sensitivity to the lectins that are found in certain foods, which makes them vulnerable to autoimmune disorders. On the other hand, those who belong to this blood group are known to present fewer risk factors for chronic conditions. In comparison to the other blood groups, they present increased physical and mental fitness. Moreover, they adapt to altitude easier, which is suggestive of their ancestry.

The weight gain is produced in those who have this blood type due to the consumption of toxic foods. Among these foods that contribute to the weight gain process, there are: corn, wheat, lentils and buckwheat. Other foods such as sesame seeds, peanuts and tomatoes are also present on the list. These foods should be eliminated from the diet, as they can have a negative influence over the metabolism. Consuming high quantities of the above-mentioned foods, a person will feel tired, retaining fluids and suffering from low blood sugar levels (these levels are at their lowest point after a person has finished eating).

If you have this blood type and you want to lose weight, you need to eliminate the foods that are bad for you and choose the right ones. In this way, not only you will lose weight but you will also stay healthy for the rest of your life. For example, you should eliminate chicken altogether, as it contains a harmful agglutinating lectin. This lectin can have harmful effects over your health – by binding to the blood antigen, it can increase the risk for cerebrovascular stroke and autoimmune disorders. Instead of chicken, you are allowed to consume other types of meat, such as mutton, rabbit, lamb, venison and goat.

Among the foods that should be included in the diet, there are: green leafy vegetables, low-fat dairy products, eggs and the meats that were already recommended below. Avoiding the toxic foods is essential and you need to learn how to replace them gradually with the ones that are beneficial, so that you can keep your weight under control and stay healthy no matter what. In terms of meat, you should also avoid consuming pork, beef or duck; shellfish (lobster, crab and shrimp) is not allowed either and turkey should only be consumed in moderate quantities. Other types of meat that you are allowed to eat include: veal, ostrich, pheasant and game. Also, be sure to avoid fowl, goose, partridge and quail.

When it comes to fish, you are allowed to consume cod, halibut, mackerel, salmon and sturgeon. As it mentioned above, you are not allowed to consume shellfish and you should also avoid the following: anchovy, octopus, eel, clams and prawns. As for the dairy products, you should concentrate on those that are low-fat. Among the recommended choices for dairy, there are: goat cheese, goat milk, mozzarella, fromage, feta, yogurt and cow milk. The dairy products that you should cross off from the list include blue cheese and American cheese. The only eggs that are allowed in the diet are those coming from hens.

In general, you are allowed to consume the majority of the fruits, with the following exceptions: coconut, pomegranate, avocado, Sharon fruit, Indian fig and starfruit. When it comes to vegetables, the dark leafy greens are definitely recommended for weight loss. The list of vegetables that you are not allowed to eat includes: artichoke, corn, olives, tomatoes, sweetcorn, pumpkin, radish and rhubarb. For eating and cooking, you are allowed to consume the following types of oils: walnut, wheat germ, flaxseed and olive. Other types of oil are forbidden and their consumptions should be avoided.

The list of nuts and seeds that you are allowed to eat includes: walnuts, pecans, macadamia nuts, flaxseed, chestnuts, Brazil nuts and almonds. On the other hand, you are not allowed to eat the following nuts and seeds: sunflower seeds, sesame seeds, poppy seeds, pistachios, pine nuts, peanuts, hazelnuts and cashew nuts. When it comes to legumes, you should avoid lentils and different types of beans, such as garbanzo and black beans. The grains and cereals that you are allowed to eat include: rice, oatmeal and quinoa. However, you should exclude the following from your diet: corn, tapioca, buckwheat, whole wheat and rye. Avoid consuming ketchup and pepper, as these are not good for your blood type. You should also eliminate distilled liquors from your daily life, including vodka, gin, rum, whiskey and brandy.

Those who belong to the blood type B group are known to gain weight also due to stress and the high levels of cortisol that occur as a response to stress. Chronic stress can also lead to a hormonal imbalance, with the body reacting in an abnormal manner to stressful situations. Apart from the weight gain, one can present difficulties when it comes to the recovery from the actual stress, suffering from disrupted sleeping patterns and daytime brain fog. The friendly bacteria in the GI tract can be disrupted, as well as the immune function be negatively affected. The wrong diet can lead to depression, thyroid problems (hypothyroidism) and insulin resistance, with high levels of stress.

It seems that there is also another problem those with this blood type present. The nitric oxide molecule, which plays an essential role in the stress response and the ability to recover from stress, is cleared more rapidly in those who present the type B antigen. It is recommended that visualization and meditation are used in order to manage the high levels of stress, obtaining the necessary physiological relief from the stress and maintaining the emotional balance.

For those who belong to this blood type, the chosen physical exercise should have a positive effect on both the mind and the body. It is recommended that the visualization and meditation are balanced with physical exercises that are more intense. Among the indicated choices for physical activity, there are: golf, tennis, martial arts, hiking and cycling.

Apart from meditation and physical exercise, those who have this blood type should go to bed early and sleep at least eight hours per night, so as to maintain a healthy circadian rhythm. Meditation can also be used at work, representing the perfect solution for relaxation when taking a break. It is also recommended that these persons use their mind on creative tasks, so as to reduce the risk of memory loss that can occur with aging.

The diet according to your blood type can help you lose the extra weight but also stay healthy from other points of view. Start making healthy choices today and soon you will see the results.

Chapter 5 – The blood type O diet

Those who have the blood type O are known as universal donors, being able to give red blood cells to anybody (due to the fact that they have both A and B antibody in the blood). Their blood type also makes them predisposed to certain medical conditions, such as stomach ulcers and disorders of the thyroid gland. The predisposition to stomach ulcers is related to the higher levels of stomach acid. However, this also means that they can digest meals that contain both fat and proteins. This is related to the fact that both alkaline phosphatase and lipoproteins are secreted in higher quantities at the level of the digestive tract.

The presence of the alkaline phosphatase and of the lipoproteins means that those who have this blood type can process the proteins from animal products in a more efficient manner. Apart from that, the problems that may appear at the level of the GI tract are easily solved and the absorption of the calcium is stimulated. The weight gain in those who have this blood type comes from the fact that the carbs that are eaten (especially those that come from grains) are easily converted into fats. Apart from that, the grains contain harmful lectins, with agglutinating properties. These attach immediately to the blood antigens, causing the flaring of the immune system and predisposing one to inflammation and auto-immune disorders.

In regard to the stress, it seems that those who belong to this blood type are set on the ancestral 'fight or flight' response, which is not as efficient as it was at the dawn of humanity. This can make a person predisposed to feelings of anger and hyperactivity; one can even reach as far as having manic episodes, due to the overall chemical imbalance. It seems that the destructive behaviors are exacerbated during periods of intense stress, depression or fatigue. It is recommended that, in order to keep the stress under control and lose weight at the same time, one eats only lean meat, with plenty of fresh fruits and vegetables. The diet of this blood type should be free of wheat or other grain sources and the intake of dairy products should be limited to a minimum, as these are known to be the source of intestinal complaints. At the same time, one must cross both alcohol and caffeine from the list. Both can increase the levels of adrenaline, which are already high in those who have this blood type.

If you want to lose weight with the blood type O diet, you need to also become physically active. Being in this blood group, there are a lot of benefits you can derive from physical exercise, especially when it comes to the health of your cardiovascular and musculo-skeletal system. Apart from the actual physical fitness, you will also benefit from the chemical release, which will reduce the risk of hyperactivity and manic episodes. The physical exercise does wonders on the activity of the neurotransmitters, providing a tonic effect for the entire body. If you want to be emotionally balanced, you need to start working out.

It is known that those who have this blood type can benefit the most from physical exercise, especially when compared to the other blood groups. It is recommended that physical exercise is performed at least three or four times per week, so as to guarantee both the physical health and the emotional balance. One of the most recommended types of physical exercise is aerobic and this should be performed for at least half an hour, three times per week. In order to avoid getting bored by physical activity, you should change the type of sport or routine on a weekly basis.

Having this blood type, you might be the kind of person who eats in a hurried manner, a mistake which can also lead to serious weight gain. Start educating yourself by eating all meals while sitting (this also includes any snacks, fruits or beverages between the meals). Learn how to chew your food thoroughly and pace yourself when eating, by putting the fork down between bites. Physical activity is recommended as a way to stop any cravings you might experience (especially for sugar) and also when you are feeling anxious (chemical release).

The blood type O diet should include different types of beans, including black and azuki, as these are highly beneficial. On the other hand, you should avoid lentils of different colors, tamarind and beans such as kidney or copper. Lean meat is allowed, with the following sources of protein being suggested for the diet: mutton, veal, lamb, beef and venison. You can also consume various types of fish, such as cod, mackerel and herring. Seafood is especially recommended, as it contains iodine and it can keep the thyroid gland functioning within normal levels. The meats that you are not allowed to eat include pork and goose, plus different types of bacon. You should also cross off caviar, catfish and octopus from the diet list, as well as the pickled herring or the smoke salmon. As you have seen, having this blood type means that the majority of the meats are digested efficiently, so there is no need to go on a vegetarian diet.

Apart from the meat, there are plenty of fresh vegetables that you can include within your diet, such as: collard greens, romaine lettuce, kale, spinach and broccoli. You should also consider consuming onions, garlic, artichokes, parsley and leeks. In order to keep your thyroid gland healthy and functioning, you should avoid eating cabbage, cauliflower and Brussel sprouts. You should also say no to shiitake mushrooms, alfalfa sprouts and fermented olives, as these can lead to inflammatory processes at the level of the GI tract. Other vegetables to be avoided include corn, eggplants and potatoes.

In regard to fruits, you should basically eat the ones that balance the acidity of the stomach, such as figs and plums. On the other hand, you should avoid those that stimulate the acid production at the level of the stomach, such as: oranges, strawberries, blackberries, melons, cantaloupes and coconut. All of these fruits stimulate the acid production and also the inflammation at the level of the GI tract, so it is for the best to avoid them.

The intake of dairy products should be limited to a minimum, as these can cause digestive complaints. However, you are allowed to consume the following dairy products in moderate quantities: feta, mozzarella, butter, farmer's cheese, goat cheese and soy milk. The consumption of eggs should be limited as well. For eating and cooking, you are allowed to use olive and flaxseed oil; other types of oil, such as cottonseed, safflower, corn and peanut should be excluded from the diet.

Wheat is the biggest no for those who have this blood type, as it causes weight gain and inflammation. However, you can consume the following in moderate quantities: rice, barley and millet. In terms of nuts and seeds, you are allowed to include walnuts and pumpkin seeds in your diet. Avoid eating cashews and peanuts and also poppy seeds. As for beverages, you are allowed to drink green tea, Seltzer water and wine, as all of these contain healthy antioxidants. Avoid, as it was already mentioned, alcohol, caffeine and black tea. Follow the recommendations made in this chapter and you will surely obtain the weight loss results you have always dreamt of. Moreover, you will feel healthy and filled with energy.

Chapter 6 – The blood type AB diet

The blood type AB is considered one of the rarest in the world, with only 5% of the general population having this particular blood type. It is also considered as the most recent blood group, having appeared due to a mixture of the blood types A and B. The people who have this blood type present the features from both blood types (A and B), such as the reduced levels of stomach acid and the ability to consume meat. However, the fact that there is not enough stomach acid in order to digest meat, also means that this is stored as fat deposits (hence the weight gain of those who have this blood type). Apart from that, they present increased sensitivity to the lectins contained in different types of food, being predisposed to more health problems than other groups.

In regard to the stress, it seems that the blood type AB also reacts by producing increased quantities of adrenaline. This is the main reason why one should avoid caffeine-based drinks and alcohol; these increase the adrenaline production and they also add to the weight gain. If you want to lose weight, you need to consume fresh green vegetables, dairy products (not all), seafood and soy products, such as tofu. The meats that have been smoked or cured are 100% forbidden – as they take a lot of time to be digested, due to the low levels of stomach acid, they increase the risk for stomach cancer. Instead, you are allowed to eat as much seafood as you wish, as it will provide you with the necessary proteins. Fish is also indicated to be included in the weight loss diet, with the following choices being the most recommended: sardines, tuna and salmon. You can also consume fresh red snapper and mahi-mahi. As it was already mentioned, you can eat certain dairy products as well, such as kefir or plain, simple yogurt. At the end of the chapter, you will find many more food recommendations for the weight loss diet, based on your blood type.

The low levels of stomach acid create the biggest problems and, if you want to avoid digestive complaints, you need to reduce the size of the meals and eat more frequently. What happens is that, due to the low levels of stomach acid, the food spends a longer time in the stomach and that can lead to digestive complaints. You also need to be extra careful when it comes to the combinations of foods you are eating. The right food choices can ensure that the levels of stomach acid are enough to metabolize the food. In regard to the correct combinations, you should avoid mixing the foods that require a longer time to be metabolized, such as proteins and starches.

Returning to the subject of stress, those who have the blood type AB are predisposed to increased levels of adrenaline as a response to a stressful situation. Apart from that, just like those who have the blood type B, the nitrous oxide is cleared more rapidly, which means that stress can lead to physical symptoms, the weight gain being one of the most obvious. It is known that the people who have this blood type also have the tendency to keep their emotions to themselves, compensating for them by overeating.

Physical exercise can help you reduce stress and obtain the necessary emotional balance. Given your blood type, you can engage in varied physical activities, alternating between those that are stimulating and those that are calming. Among the recommended physical activities for weight loss, you can find the following: aerobic, running, biking, yoga and Tai chi. You should practice a sport, at least two times per week, for approximately one hour. Also, you can use physical exercise during the workday, in order to feel more energized.

As with the other blood types, there are specific food recommendations to be made for the blood type AB. When it comes to meat, you are allowed to eat lamb, mutton, rabbit and turkey. On the other hand, you should avoid the following meats: pork (bacon, ham), beef (steak, ground), chicken, duck, goose, veal, venison and buffalo. In terms of seafood, you are recommended to eat the following: albacore, cod, mackerel, mahi-mahi, pike, rainbow trout, red snapper, sailfish, sardine, sea trout, snail and surgeon. Even though seafood is highly beneficial for those who have this blood type, there are certain produce you should avoid, such as: anchovy, beluga, clam, crab, crayfish, eel, halibut, herring, lobster, smoked salmon, oyster and shrimp.

Apart from yogurt and kefir, these are the other dairy products you are allowed to consume: cottage cheese, sour cream, ricotta, mozzarella, goat milk, goat cheese and feta. Among the dairy products that you need to cross off from the list, there are: parmesan, brie, blue cheese and American cheese. You should need to avoid whole milk, butter and buttermilk, as well as ice cream and sherbet. For eating and cooking, you are allowed to use olive oil and, if you want, cod liver, flaxseed or peanut oil. On the other hand, these are the types of oil that you should eliminate from your diet: sunflower, sesame, safflower, cottonseed and corn.

The nuts and seeds that you are allowed to include in your diet are: chestnuts, peanuts (including peanut butter) and walnuts. You should avoid filbert nuts and the following seeds: sunflower, sesame, pumpkin and poppy. Tahini and sunflower butter should be excluded from the diet. In terms of beans and legumes, you should include the following in your diet: beans (soy, red, pinto and navy) and green lentils. The other types of beans – lima, kidney, garbanzo, fava, black, azuki and aduke – should be excluded from the list, as well as the black eyed peas.

When it comes to cereals, you should add these to your diet: millet, oat, bran, oatmeal, rice bran, puffed rice, ryeberry and spelt. Avoid the following cereals, as these are not beneficial for your body: buckwheat, cornflakes, cornmeal, kamut and kasha. In terms of other grains, you are allowed to eat: brown rice bread, rice cakes, rye bread, soy flour bread and sprouted wheat bread. Be sure to avoid the corn muffins, as these contribute to the weight gain process. You can also benefit from the products that are made or contain the following types of flour: oat, rice, rye and sprouted wheat. Include different types of rice in your diet, including basmati, brown, white and wild rice in your diet but avoid the following choices: soba noodles, artichoke pasta, barley flour and buckwheat kasha.

The list of vegetables you are allowed to include in your diet is quite long, including: yams, alfalfa sprouts, sweet potatoes, garlic, kale, eggplant, collard greens, cucumbers, celery, cauliflower, broccoli and beets. There are certain vegetables that you should avoid, such as: peppers, radishes, black olives, corn, avocado and artichokes. As for fruits, you have some pretty varied choices here available as well: plums, lemons, pineapple, grapefruit, grapes, kiwi, figs, cherries and cranberries. The fruits that you are not allowed to eat include: starfruit, rhubarb, pears, pomegranates, oranges, mangoes, guava, coconuts and bananas. You can also consume fresh juices made from these fruits but make sure that you avoid the orange juice.

In terms of beverages, you are allowed to consume green tea, as it contains healthy antioxidants. The list of beverages that you should exclude from your diet includes: caffeine-based beverages, black tea, distilled liquors (vodka, rum, gin, whiskey, brandy) and sugary drinks (including diet soda). Condiments should be excluded from the diet as well, especially the following ones: pickles, relish, ketchup and Worcestershire sauce. Organize your list with what you are allowed to eat and what you should exclude from the diet, so as to guarantee the weight loss results on a long-term basis.

Conclusion

I hope this book was able to provide information on how to lose weight in a healthy manner, with the blood type diet.

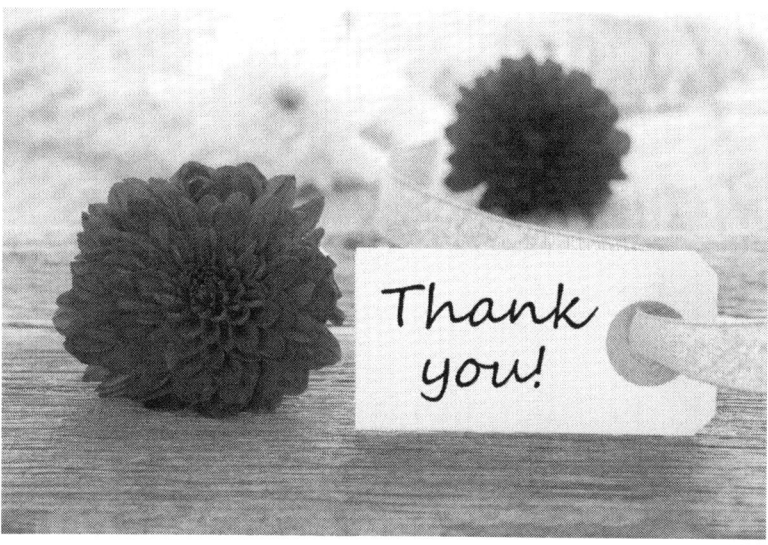

Finally, if you enjoyed this book, then I'd like to ask you for a favor, would you be kind enough to leave a review for this book on Amazon? It'd be greatly appreciated!

Thank you and good luck!

Made in the USA
San Bernardino, CA
14 December 2015